The Magic of Salt

To Heal and for Beauty

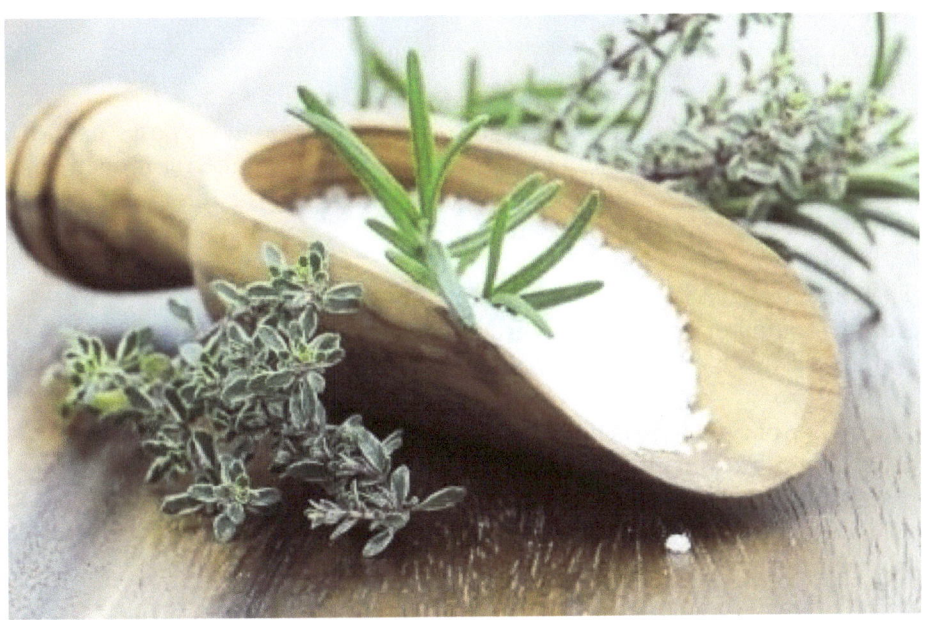

Dueep J Singh

Natural Remedy Series

Mendon Cottage Books

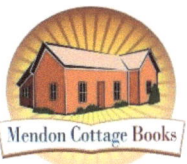

JD-Biz Publishing

Disclaimer

The information is this book is provided for informational purposes only. It is not intended to be used and medical advice or a substitute for proper medical treatment by a qualified health care provider. The information is believed to be accurate as presented based on research by the author.

The contents have not been evaluated by the U.S. Food and Drug Administration or any other Government or Health Organization and the contents in this book are not to be used to treat cure or prevent disease.

The author or publisher is not responsible for the use or safety of any diet, procedure or treatment mentioned in this book. The author or publisher is not responsible for errors or omissions that may exist.

Warning

The Book is for informational purposes only and before taking on any diet, treatment or medical procedure, it is recommended to consult with your primary health care provider.

Our books are available at

1. Amazon.com

2. Barnes and Noble

3. Itunes

4. Kobo

5. Smashwords

6. Google Play Books

Table of Contents

Introduction

In this book, you are going to know more about the power of a very common ingredient, found in every one's kitchen. This is salt, without which any salty dish is going to lose its savor and flavor.

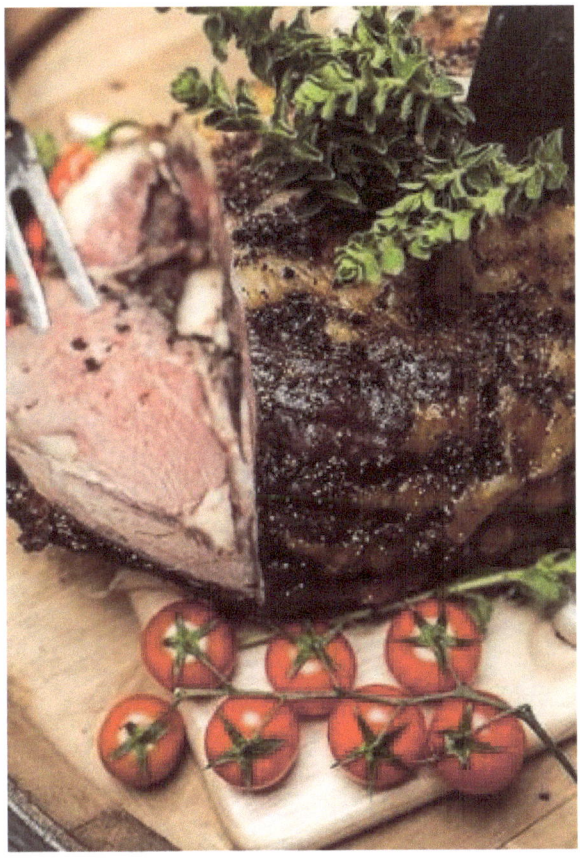

Imagine food without salt!

Salt was held to be so precious in ancient times, that Roman soldiers were given salt daily at night, as salary. The idea was that they were going to have enough of salt in which they could cook their evening meal, with ground corn and onions. This was the diet on which the Roman legions marched and conquered half of the world. More than 3000 years ago, salt was used as a coin to ransom Kings and conquered prisoners, along with spices, which were considered to be more precious than precious stones and gold.

It is a historically known fact that Portuguese, German and British rulers of Africa asked the local chieftains to pay their taxes in ivory, local produce, and salt. That is the reason why, the idea of "he eats salt with his food," was said to describe a rich man. Even as late as the 19th century, when the transport system had improved imports of salt to Africa, the fierce warriors in innermost Africa still demanded salt from and of their conquered prisoners. The average man did not have salt to eat, and that is why he flavored his food with aromatic leaves and other herbs gathered from the forests.

It is also a historical fact that the British tried out the same idea of taxation on salt in India, and that immediately brought the whole of India United up in arms, in their fight for independence. Salt was the birthright of every poor person in India, and putting the tax on salt was almost as much a tyranny, as putting tax on something like say, water or the air one breathed. The whole of India joined in the fight for independence, because they did not want rulers, who wanted to tax the salt they ate in their food. The quit India movement thus gained more popularity and impetus. And that is one of the factors which may be British decide to quit India in 1947.

Ancient medical treatises in Egypt and Persia considered salt to be necessary ingredient in making up nostrums and remedies to cure ills. Also, salt was used as a scrub, instead of soap or even sand, to remove dust and grime after a hard days work. In many religious ceremonies, salt was considered to be with the most pure of ingredients, and that is why it was offered to the gods.

If you go to Russia, you are going to be welcomed with the bread and salt. This has a historical significance. The idea of eating one's salt, and being loyal to one's salt has come down through millenniums, as the way in which feudal lords managed to keep the loyalty of the people under them. The one who had betrayed his own salt was a traitor to whom nobody would give any welcome.

The underlying significance was a soldier worked for a feudal lord. He was paid enough with which he could afford to buy precious salt for his food. Even today in the East, one takes the pinch of salt offered to him by a friend, or by an acquaintance, to acknowledge that his loyalty remains with the friend who has made him a brother of the salt.

This tradition of bread and salt offered to guests meant that the doors of the host were open. They would be given bread, to sustain them. The food would be seasoned by salt and once that salt was eaten, the guest was honorbound to abide by the rules of honor and friendship to protect the family and the lands of the host, when required.

You may remember a childhood fairytale, called Ali Baba and the 40 thieves. In the original story, the loyal and intelligent slave girl Marjiana got suspicious of the thief chieftain hunting for his treasure, when he came to Ali Baba's house disguised as a merchant with 40 barrels – jars of oil. When asked to stay for dinner, he said "I have made a vow, that I shall not eat bread and salt, for all those days which it will take me to reach my destination, and sell my barrels of oil profitably and successfully. "

The simple and good Ali Baba took this vow for something done by a pious man. The more worldly Marjiana's suspicions are immediately aroused by this phrase, eating bread and salt. That immediately meant that the new guest in their house meant harm to the family and to her master. And so she used the classic method of pouring boiling oil into all the oil jars and killed the 40 thieves.

Production Of Salt

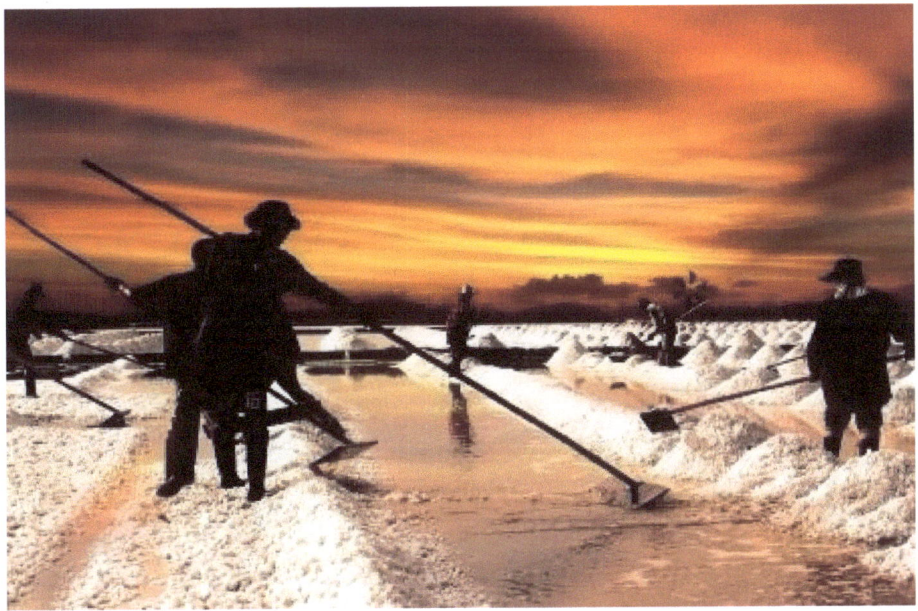

Salt is one of the many natural products in Nature, of which she has unlimited resources. As long as there is seawater or Lake water somewhere on the surface of the earth, you are going to get salt.

This once precious and loyalty causing salt was obtained from salt water, which normally was found after one evaporated salt water on the beaches in shallow troughs.

There are beaches all over the world, where you can find piles of salt, just drying out in the sun. This salt is going to have a lot of impurities in it, because after all the seawater brought with it seaweed and other items from the sea. This salt is collected and sent to factories, where it is powdered, and purified.

In India, and in other parts of the East, they have begun adding iodine to the salt, to prevent thyroid and goiter problems. But then, they could always use the seaweed from the sea, to get pure iodine.

Salt is not limited to salt water; you can find it on land too, especially in salt beds, where once seas existed. The upheavals in the land masses, brought about 7000 years ago made plenty of seas dry while in other places, mountains like the Himalayas came up, where there was once plain land. In fact, you can find fossils of fishes in the Himalayas, which may also lead one to think that it is very easy for one to find salt beds there, if only one has the inclination to dig in the snow.

One of these areas in the Indian subcontinent, which was once under the Tethys Ocean millenniums ago is now land with some desert area. This desert in India is called theThar Desert. You have salt beds here, where crystallized salt formed by the drying of the sea, ages ago, cover the surface of the desert. In the same way, you have desert and dry areas in the USA – California, Illinois, Ohio-and Canada, where you can get these salt beds.

This salt is not limited to just seawater. Dried lakes have also given rise to salt sea beds. Nevertheless, you are going to get these ancient salt sea beds in places all over the world, ranging from Africa, Siberia, Asia and the USA to places in Europe where salt sea beds are being discovered by people following wild or domesticated animals going to their favorite "salt lick". That was how salt was found in the Thar desert ages ago, when deer were found going every morning to a place to lick the ground.

So it should not be surprising, that when Alexander came to India to conquer the area of Sind, more than 3000 years ago, his horses found an amazing salt lick by the sides of the mountains. It seems that sick horses got miraculously rejuvenated, after they had licked a dose of this healthy, rocksalt, over a given period of time. That is why the keepers of the horses in Alexander's army requested him to make temporary stables for their horses, near the Salt Lick.

His soldiers were extremely thrilled too. Here they were with unlimited treasure, right in front of their eyes, when previously, they were given out, measured out doles of salt, every evening by their officers. Most of them decided not to go back to Greece. Instead, they settle down there in that area, and decided to raise their own families. That is why people of the Northwest Frontier region of the Indian subcontinent have Grecian /Caucasian features, and are extremely fair with gray, blue and green eyes and light colored hair.

This area where this salt is extracted from the earth is known as Khivra – now in Pakistan – and for 3000 years, it has been mined extensively, with no end in sight.

My father knew people who lived in that area, for centuries, and one of them described the mines of Khivra to my 10-year-old father. The imagery of long mine shafts, with transparent mirrorlike salt deposits going what looked like miles and miles going into the interior of underground mines would be fascinating to any child.

These mines sent salt to local areas and to other parts of India and other countries in the East, as rock salt for centuries. They were put under British management in the 18th century, when this salt began to be exported by sea to Europe as a seasoning for food and a health giving spice.

This rock salt – also known all over the world as Sendha Namak- is normally pink in color, and is considered to be the best and purest ingredient to make up natural remedies, since ancient times. Along with rock salt, you are also going to get black salt – called Kala Namak-on- land.

Black salt, like rock salt is milder in taste than sea salt and has a spicier taste. This salt can also be found in salt beds, especially in the Scandinavian countries.

Differentiate between Rock Salt And Black Salt

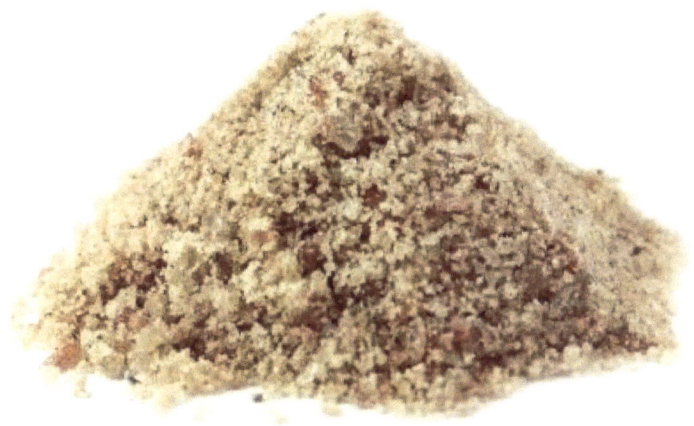

Black salt of South Asia

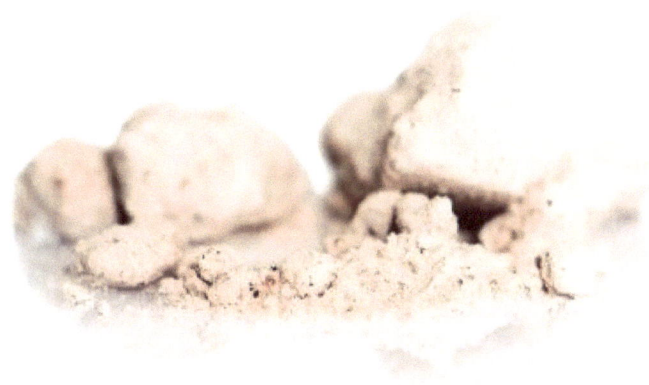

It can also be in this form

Rock salt looks like these crystals...

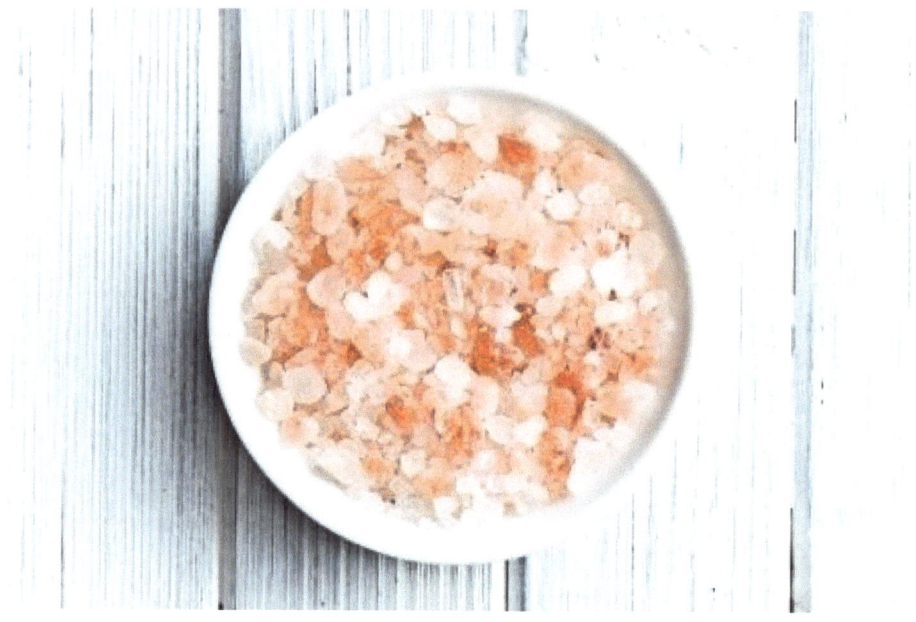

How are you going to differentiate between rock salt and black salt? Firstly, rocksalt is more of a crystalline salt. It is going to be in a variety of colors, ranging from white to pink and even pale yellow, and it is not going to have a very strong aroma. On the other hand, black salt has a very distinct aroma. It almost reminds one of rotten eggs.

This black salt is considered to be an extremely delicious and spicy additive to Eastern cuisine, especially when you are making snacks and spicy dishes. Salads, chopped fruit and vegetables are sprinkled with black salt, pepper and roasted cumin seeds to give them that extra spicy touch.

Rock salt is a more healthier substitute, for common sea salt, when you are preparing meals for your family. In fact, the sea salt you get in the East is so heavily iodized, and processed, that we do not know the additives put in them. That is why I go to my friendly neighborhood grocers'and ask him for a chunk of rock salt. That is because I live in an area, where it is very easy for me to get rock salt. I grind it up in my own grinder, and there I am, I have this fine powder, which is going to be used to cook delicious meals and healthy dishes for the family.

In the same way, I can always ask him for a chunk of black salt. Black salt can be anywhere between Brown to black in color. That is because the sulfate and sulfide content in this salt is more. Ordinary sea salt has more of sodium and chloride in it. When I grind this, this is also going to make up a pinkish dark brown powder.

I easily know the difference between rock salt and black salt, just by giving the glass jars a hearty sniff. Anything which smells stronger is definitely black salt. Good for digestion, and good to add a spicy je ne sais quoi of piquancy to any salad, salad dressing, fruit and vegetable mixture, lightly fried sprouts mixture, or anything other healthy light snack I want to enjoy between meals.

How Harmful Is Salt Really?

Believe it or not, so many people have been scared by doctors who have brought scientific proof in front of them, that salt is extremely harmful to their health, that they have stopped eating salty food altogether. In some ways, the doctors are right, because processed foods have high quantity of salt added. So if you are not eating processed foods, in your daily diet, **do not stop eating salt.**

Your body needs anywhere between ½ teaspoon to 1 ½ teaspoon of salt, throughout the day in all your meals. That is because it is an essential mineral to keep your body functioning properly. However, we have this bad habit of sprinkling extra salt all over our meals, and that is the reason why our salt intake increases. And our doctor says that we need to reduce salt in our diet.

What happens then? We go overboard. We stop eating salt altogether. The body demands salt, but it is not getting it. It goes into drastic action mode. It starts getting rid of excess of water in the body. We are very happy, because we think that we have lost weight. After that, it starts preserving the remaining amount of salt in the body. Because after all, the show must go on, and the body needs to function properly. The body starts to swell up.

We go back to our doctor. He says hmmmm hmmmm pensively, asks us to undergo some more tests because he really cannot make out why there is water retention in the body, and then prescribes some expensive chemical-based drugs for us.

You could have saved all this, by just reducing your salt intake, from 1 teaspoon in the whole day, to say, ¾ teaspoon. At least your body would be getting some salt, would not it.

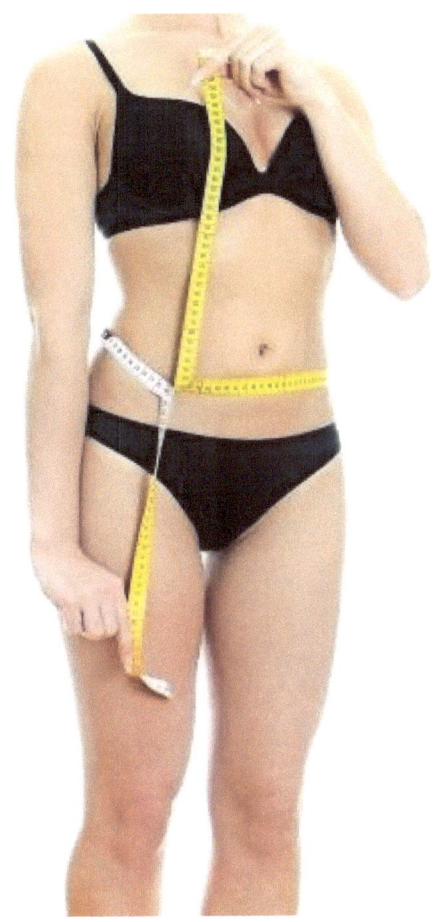

Will I lose weight, if I cut salt completely out of my diet?

If you think that removing salt and sugar from your diet is going to help you lose weight, think again. You may go in for dietetic products, but you are just paying a high price and premium for these special foods. You are paying for these companies not to add sugar, as well as salt to your processed special reproducing foods. So that means you are paying more money for less goods.

If you want the best diet foods, make them yourself. Make sure that they do have some sugar and some rock salt in them. Cutting sugar and salt totally out of your diet is definitely not recommended.

Salt for Common Ailments

Salt was used in small quantities by ancient sages and medicine men to make up ancient medical remedies. All they needed to do was collect a handful of salt, pound it and use pinches of it in different brews, lotions, potions and concoctions. Countries in the east never had a dearth of salt, because they were near to the sea. It was only landlocked areas where salt was considered precious.

So as salt was as common and easily available as fresh water in the East, medicines using salt as one of the ingredients were extremely common. Ancient Chinese, Japanese, Egyptian, Mesopotamian, Greek and Indian medicine men used plenty of salt as it was considered to be a purifier.

Sea salt and rocksalt was considered to be anti-bileous, anti-phlegmatic and also anti-aciditic in nature. Being natural products, these salts were easily absorbed in the body and got the system moving. That is the reason why since ancient times, every religious ceremony in the East consisted of purifying religious dishes flavored with rocksalt. Even in Egyptian, ancient Greek, Roman, Persian and Babylonian tradition, the priests began their worship of the gods by making up a mixture of incense, spices, flowers and salt.

So here are some extremely easy to follow recipes, which you would want to use, to cure you of common ailments.

Buttermilk

1 pint unsweetened yogurt.

1 pint water along with ice cubes

four – six mint leaves

Rock salt /black salt/pepper to taste

Roasted cumin seeds – powdered

Mix yogurt, ice cubes, water, mint leaves, spices and cumin seeds in your blender, and blend until frothy. Serve in tall glasses with more powdered cumin seeds, chopped mint leaves and pepper.

This can also be drunk sweet when it is made with honey – that is going to take a little more time, because honey does not dissolve very easily in this cold mixture – but this is considered to be the best digestive and refreshing drink available to you of a hot summer. You can also drink this with your lunch, to make sure that your meal is digested properly.

Summertime is definitely not the time to eat heavy meals. Nevertheless, people, especially in the north of India cannot resist heavy meals during summer, especially when they are leafy spinach with cornbread. This is totally indigestible, but when it is drunk with spiced buttermilk, it is digested easily. Besides this, the sedentary lifestyle is not so very common in many backwaters of the East, where people slog in hard physical labor from dawn to dusk, in order to survive or eke out a meager living. So if they manage to get to drink buttermilk, they are always going to salt it well.

This salt prevents a body from getting dehydrated when it has to work outdoors in all weathers.

You may ask why I placed buttermilk under the heading of salt for common ailments. That is because many of the herbal cures given here used since ancient times call for buttermilk.

Diarrhea

In ancient times, when people did not know much about chemical-based artificially manufactured drugs – the bane of technological development – they used ancient remedies with which they could keep their families healthy. Diarrhea was a very common ailment, especially when they did not bother much about keeping their fruit and vegetables clean before eating. Also, they did not bother much about elementary hygiene like washing one's hands before eating something. So the moment somebody fell victim to diarrhea. He was immediately fed buttermilk with a little rock salt.

This was given to him with food or after food. This light food was called "khichri" or kedgeree as it is called in 20th century Brit cuisine.

Recipe for Khichri – kedgeree

The rock salt, which is added to this dish – easily digestible and amazingly good for invalid food – aids the food to get digested easily, while adding the salty, spicy content to a mixture of rice and lentils.

INGREDIENTS:

Khichri

1/2 Cup - Yellow or green Moong Dal [This is the Dal- lentil, bean- which is normally used to make bean sprouts.]
1 Cup Basmati Rice
To Taste - Rock Salt/black salt and pepper along with powdered roasted cumin seeds, sprinkled on top of the dish.
5-6 Cups - Water
For Tadka/seasoning
2 Tsp - Ghee/Oil

3-4 - Green Chili

A Pinch - Asafoetida/Hing

1 tsp - Cumin Seeds/Jeera

2 tsp - Minced Garlic

METHOD:

Clean the rice as well as the mung and then soak it for 15 minutes. Add three cups water to the rice and the dal and allow to cook till the water is absorbed. If you have a pressure cooker, allow it to whistle thrice. That means that this is going to be cooked into porridge consistency.

It takes a while for green mung to be cooked, so you may soak it overnight. If you think that the water has been absorbed, and the rice and the dal has not quite reach the porridge consistency, you can add some more water. This quantity is going to depend on how watery or how thick you want your porridge to be.

If you are going to be using it as comfort food, you can do the tempering. If you are going to be using it as food for invalids, just add rock salt, pepper and a little bit of lemon juice sprinkled on top, and give it to your patient with a bowl of yogurt. This is easy to digest.

Tempering is what is going to give that extra touch of yumminess to this Khichdi.

Mix the garlic with the cumin seeds and chop the chilies. Heat the oil in your frying pan, add garlic and asafoetida and fry until it is a Golden brown. Now add the chilies and fry until you hear the crackle of the seeds. Fry this on low heat, because fried chilies are quite capable of making your eyes water, because of their strong smell, which seems to be enhanced by a little bit of frying in oil.

Now spread this tempering all over the rice and serve boiling hot.

Flatulence

Grind some onions, which you may use for cooking. Preserve the onion water. Sprinkle rocksalt on this onion water, and drink it up. This is considered to be the best remedy to save you from flatulence.

You may also want to try drinking one teaspoonful of ginger juice, with a little bit of rock salt half an hour before you eat a meal. Not only is this going to improve your digestion, but it prevents indigestion, constipation, and also flatulence.

Headache / Migraine

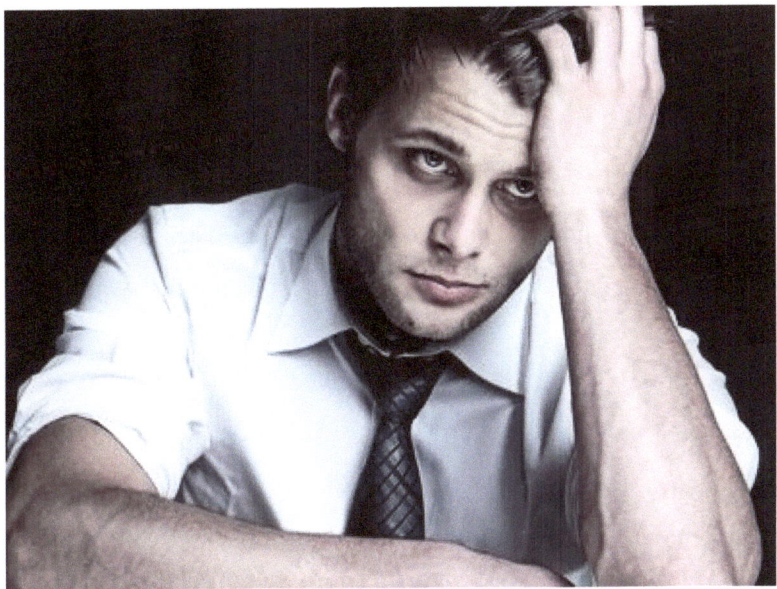

Did you know that you can get rid of headaches very easily, just by putting one drop of salt water in your nostrils. I saw an old naturopath using an eyedropper to do just that and get rid of his headaches. I have a feeling, that that made him sneeze, so if the headache was due to some nasal congestion, or blockage, well, that got rid of the cause of the headache. Also, he told me to put a Pinch of rocksalt on my tongue and allow it to dissolve for 10 minutes, before I swallow the salty saliva down with ice cold water. I guess, this idea was to make sure that if I was suffering from a dehydration headache, I got the necessary amounts of salt and water into my system!

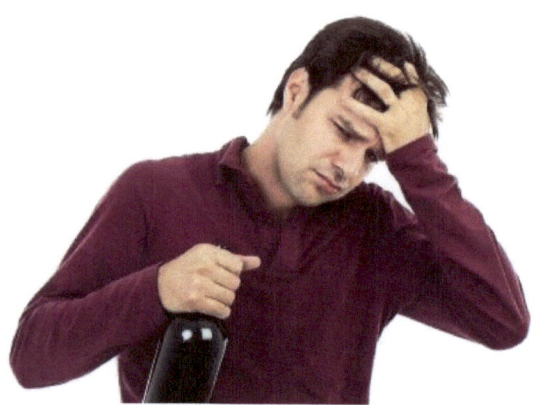

Less water in your body brought about by dehydration or by drinking can also cause a headache, apart from a hangover…

In the same way, if you are suffering from **migraine**, you may try this migraine remedy. Add half a teaspoonful of salt to half a teaspoonful of honey. This may help to alleviate the pain. I did not know about this remedy, when I used to suffer from migraine up to my 40s, but then any sort of knowledge is always useful. Besides, it is well-known that migraine attacks disappear as a person grows older.

Dandruff Elimination

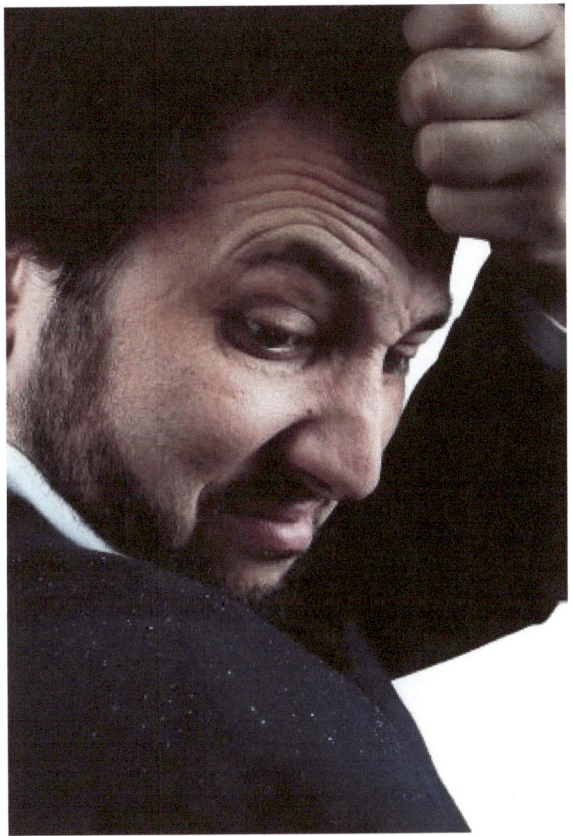

Oooops, dandruff! So very embarrassing…

I have been to many villages where salt is still being used as a way to get rid of dandruff. You may have noticed that many companies out there selling you dandruff relieving products are going to use this advertising copy, "keep your hair dandruff free for a week by using our special dandruff shampoo." *What they are definitely not going to tell you is that in most and mild cases it takes seven days for the dandruff flakes to accumulate on your scalp.* They are just dried skin cells of the epidermis on your scalp. So on the seventh day, you wash your head with the shampoo, and are really pleased, because all the flakes are gone.

Instead, if you had washed your hair with water in which you had added 3 tablespoons of salt and 1 tablespoon of olive or coconut oil, you would never have been bothered by dandruff ever. So if you are suffering from a serious case of dandruff, you may try this natural remedy for keeping your scalp healthy.

Dandruff Removal Oil

Warm-up one teaspoonful of salt in half a cup of your favorite scalp massage oil, which can be coconut, olive, or any other moisturising oil you prefer. You may also add the juice of half a lemon. Rub this early in your scalp, and allow the salt and the oil to soak into the skin for half an hour. Now shampoo with a mild shampoo. You may use a natural herbal shampoo, or you may make up an **egg shampoo**, by mixing the yolk of an egg with 1 tablespoon full of powdered Fullers Earth. This shampoo is considered to be the best way in which people in the East got all the dust and grime out of their hair, for centuries.

Taking Care of Tooth Trouble

Did you know that apart from clove oils, salt was the best way in which you could keep tooth trouble, tooth decay and tooth pain at bay. So is it surprising, that oldsters long ago, always made sure that they rinsed their mouth regularly after every meal with saltwater. Also, they made sure that the "toothpaste" with which they brushed their teeth twice a day was made up of a mixture of mustard oil with three teaspoonfuls of rocksalt and placed in the sun for a day to ripen. This prevented gingivitis and infected gums.

Of course, the brushes that they used were made up of neem twigs, but as we do not enjoy chewing on bitter green twigs, brushing our teeth with them, and so cleaning our dental set, we can always use a finger to brush and massage our teeth and gums with this salt toothpaste.

Cold and Cough Remedy

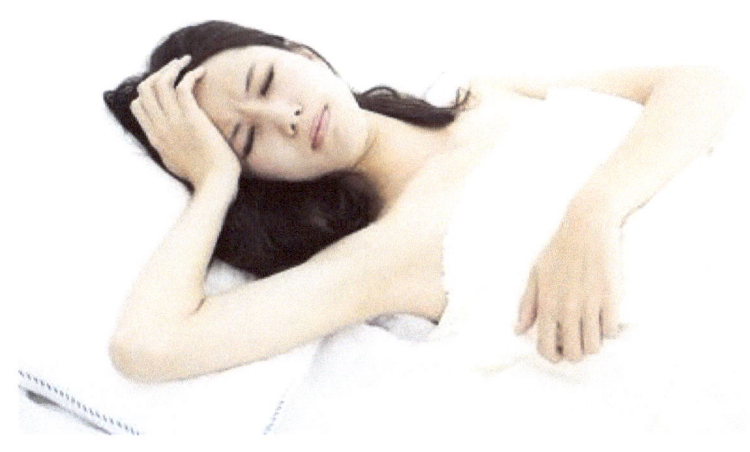

A cold may leave you feeling feverish and headachy

If you are suffering from a cold, add ground five black peppercorns, 1/8 teaspoonful of rock salt and two pinches of turmeric. Boil them together in one glass of water. Sip this slowly. This is going to help in curing your cold.

It ticklish cough can be alleviated by sucking on a rock salt crystal. I found that rock candy also does the same thing – moisturizes the throat and prevents it from drying.

Gargle with salt water, and also rinse your nostrils with saltwater – 1/8 teaspoonful of salt in a glass of warm water thrice a day, to get rid of any sort of hoarseness, infection and cold related problems.

Salt Fomentation

Salt has been used since ancient times as an excellent fomentation medium. I saw an athlete trainer asking one of his athletes to do this fomentation to reduce the swelling, brought about by sprains, and bruises, which are so much a part of an athlete's training program.

How do you make a salt fomentation bag? Heat some salt on a griddle pan. Add a little bit of oil to this salt. Now place all of this heated salt into a muslin cloth and make up a small bag. Place it toward the effective area.

You may also want to massage that area with a ghee and salt mixture. This gives you relief from pain. This is also going to eliminate any sort of swelling really soon.

No wonder I see so many of my athlete friends, who prepare salt fomentation bags beforehand. Whenever they find themselves facing bruises and strains, all they have to do is use these bags, instead of hot water bottles. They just heat up the griddle pan and then take it off the fire, to allow it to cool from really hot to pleasantly hot. They then place the bags on that griddle and allow the salt to absorb the heat. Of course, this has to be heated every 15 to 20 minutes, but it is considered to be the most effective swelling relief remedy.

Bronchitis Relief

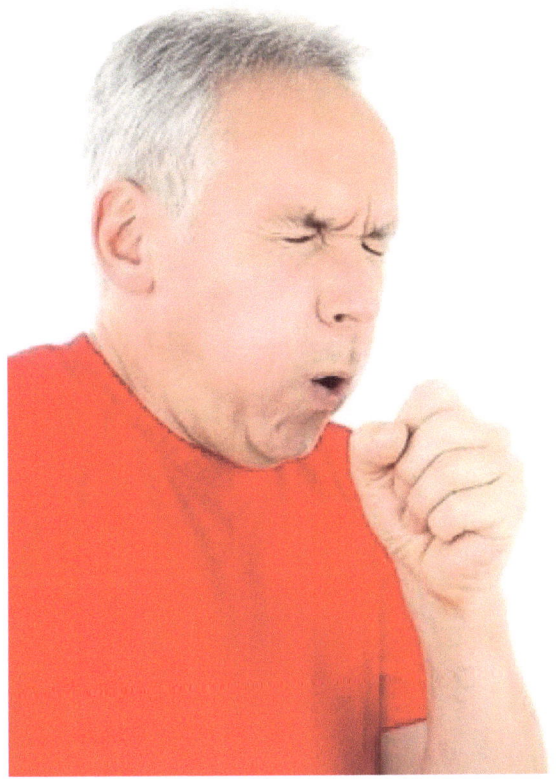

This salt –ghee massage can also be done for people suffering from bronchitis by massaging the affected areas with one warm teaspoonful of this mixture. Do this once a day.

Arthritis relief

If you have somebody in the family suffering from arthritis, and you have salt nearby,well, you do not have to worry. Foment the affected area with salted hot water, in a hot water bottle. You are going to find relief from joint pain. You can also massage that affected area with arthritis oil.

Traditional arthritis oil

This arthritis oil can be used, especially in the winter, when you are suffering from aching joints. It is also effective in giving you relief from sprains.

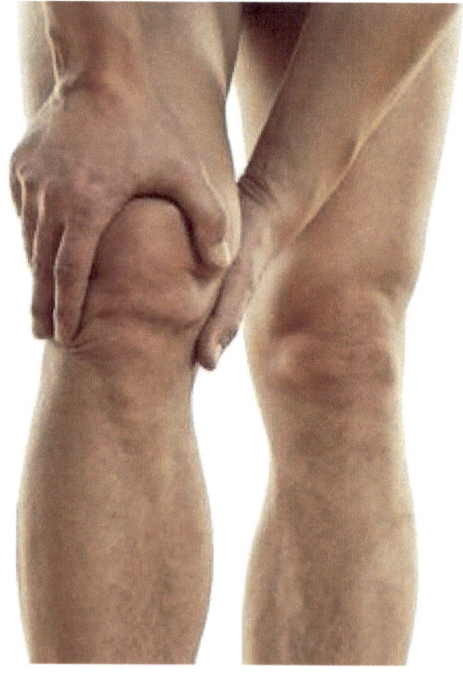

This oil is very strong, and that is why it has to be used in small quantities. That is because it uses unrefined mustard oil as the base. This is considered to be one of the best oils in the East to prevent or heal joint problems, sprains, and make the joints more supple in arthritis.

Take half a bottle of mustard oil. To this, add 2 teaspoons full of salt, ¼ teaspoonful of cayenne pepper, half a teaspoonful of ground ginger powder and 2 powdered cloves and mix well. Place this powerful arthritis oil in a glass bottle. Allow it to bake in the sun for one day. Once you have made this mixture, you can always use it throughout the winter to get relief from joint ache, sprains and other joint and muscle related problems.

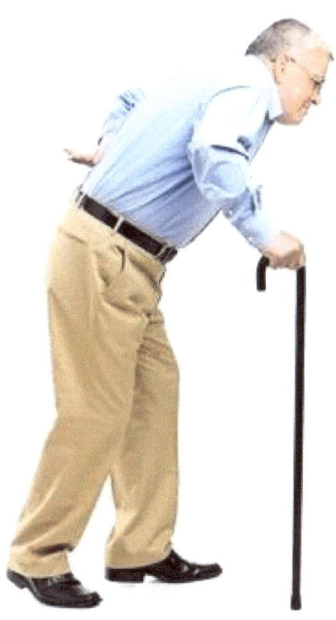

No joint pain or back pain, thanks to regular massages with this traditional arthritis oil

Remember that cayenne is going to sting when it comes in contact with skin. So use this in small quantities. Massage twice a day, with the patient sitting in the sun.

Salt for Beauty

Salt has been used for millenniums as a natural beauty rub by beauties of every civilization known to mankind. Salt is an excellent skin exfoliater, getting rid of all the dry dead cells on your skin. So you may want to add sea salt to your bath to prevent skin diseases, get rid of the dirt and grime and also to feel refreshed.

Sea Salt Scrub

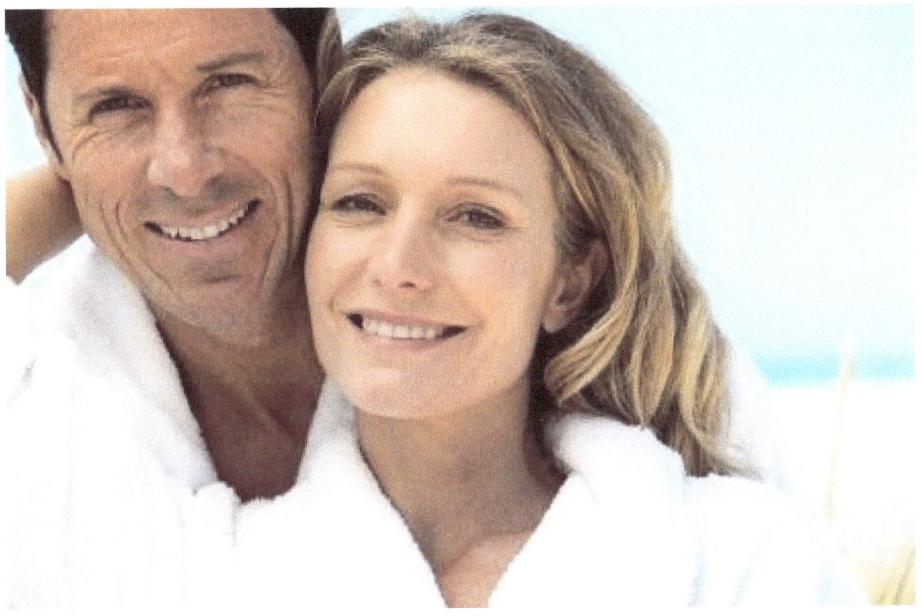

If you are down by the sea, take full advantage of saltwater baths and sea salt scrubs.

You can either make a sea salt scrub by rubbing yourself briskly with pure sea salt before you have a shower. That is, of course, the way in which the ancients had a bath, because they believed that salt was the purest of natural ingredients. That is why they wetted the salt and then rubbed this half wet mixture gently all over the surface of their skins. After that, they went right into the water and allowed the salt to take with it the dust and the grime accumulated during the day's work.

Skin problems

You can also get rid of skin problems by massaging your body with warm olive oil in which you have added half a teaspoonful of salt. You may want to add a drop of your preferred essential oil to this mixture in order to give it a mild perfume.

Pimples and acne

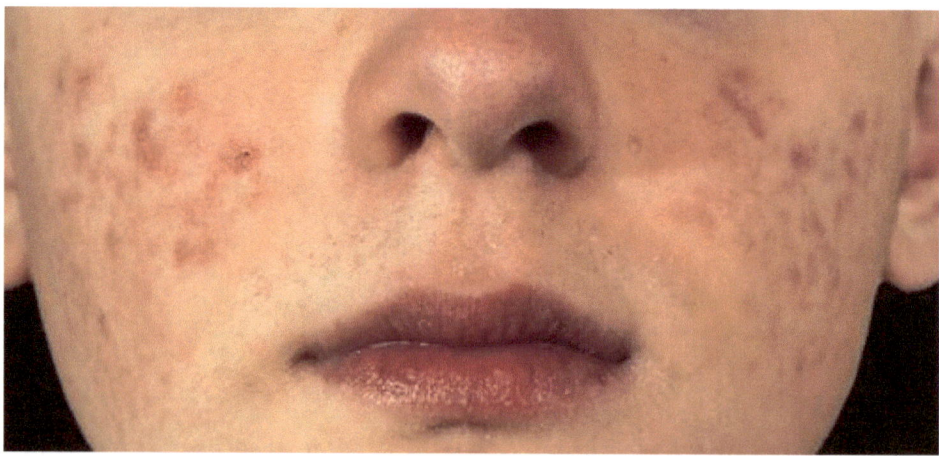

If you are suffering from acne and pimples, all you have to do is to add a little rock salt to half a teaspoonful of ginger juice. Apply this mixture to all the affected areas. The rock salt is an antiseptic and is going to cure the acne. The ginger juice is a powerful curative, which is going to promote the growth of the infected cells and prevent further infection.

Prickly heat

Are you suffering from prickly heat? This normally takes up the form of small eruptions on the surface of your skin, especially if the atmosphere is moist muggy, as well as hot. Try drinking lots of fruit juice with lots of rock salt, black pepper and lemon juice. Not only is this going to cool down your system, but it is also going to leave your skin glowing and blemish free.

Skin Moisturizer for Itching

If your skin is itching, just make a scrub with 1 tablespoon wheat bran, half a teaspoonful of rock salt, one teaspoonful of honey and 1 teaspoon olive oil. Apply this all over the affected areas. This is immediately going to stop any set of itching or possible skin problems brought about exposure to the sun, the summer, a dehydrated skin or any other factors.

Eczema Cure

Salt water is of course the best way in which you can prevent and cure. Simple skin problems, including eczema, which latter can also be cured by rubbing the affected area with turpentine, and rocksalt until you are cured.

Fungal skin infection cure

Now this is one cure, which I found out for myself. I found a patch of dark discolored skin in between my fingers, – this was not athletes foot – some weeks ago. It definitely did not itch, so I considered this to be a reaction from dishwashing powder chemicals or perhaps a local fungal infection. Neither did it spread.

I cured it completely by mixing 1 teaspoon each of glycerin, Neem Oil, salt and rubbing alcohol [the one used to clean the surface of your skin, before the doctor injects you with a hypodermic.]

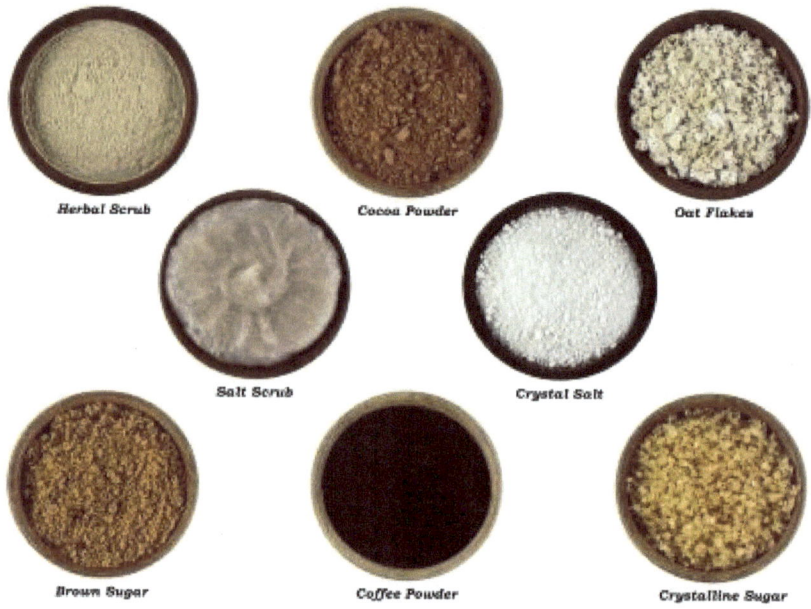

Herbal Scrub   Cocoa Powder   Oat Flakes

Salt Scrub   Crystal Salt

Brown Sugar   Coffee Powder   Crystalline Sugar

Natural Ingredients to keep you beautiful!

I knew that the alcohol would dry up that skin area, the glycerin would keep it moisturized, the neem oil, and the salt would cure it. I rubbed this morning and evening, and it disappeared within 3 to 4 days. My skin is now back to normal. I do not know what it was, but remember that salt is a powerful antiseptic, so you can use it to cure mild cuts and wounds washed in saline water and then bandaged after an antiseptic is placed on them. Doctors do it, so can you.

I remember the story of a very brave soldier, whose ship was shelled during the Second World War. He was badly burned, and he managed to keep afloat, half submerged in the sea for two days, before he was picked up. The doctors were extremely surprised to see that he did not suffer from any infection, resulting from those serious burns and wondered how that came about. "Waal," he drawled in a laconic tone, " I guess,I have been soaking all those injured areas in salt water for the past two days."

So I wonder why doctors do not use the saltwater cure to cure burns?

Where Do You Buy Rock Salt/Black Salt?

I am not very certain about the quality of the powdered rock salt, which you may find on Amazon.com or on eBay. There are companies talking about pure powdered rocksalt, but I would not be surprised if most of this salt is going to be a mixture of ordinary salt, a little bit of rock salt to give it the pinkish tint, and even a little bit of finely ground chalk powder. [Yes, heard of a company somewhere in the world doing that.]

So I would suggest that you look for a place where you can get pure rocksalt crystals. If you are in the East, you can always get rocksalt crystals or lumps of black salt in shops nearby, because they are a necessary part of eastern cuisine and medicine.

If you are in the West, you would want to get them from a proper and reputed dealer in the East. Look for a shop, with a good reputation and plenty of reviews. Look for the best deals they are going to give you. Also look at shipping time.

Bargains are available all over the world, especially in the East. Negotiate. Rock Salt is not so precious that you need to pay a king's ransom for 10 g of salt. I was astonished to see people paying anywhere between EUR15-EUR20 for 10 g of powdered rocksalt. Well, they would rather pay this exorbitant amount, instead of going online, and looking for places where they could get a pound of rocksalt crystals with shipping charges added – anywhere between USD5-USD10!

So if you are really concerned about your health, do a little bit of online research right now.

Salt in Your Cuisine

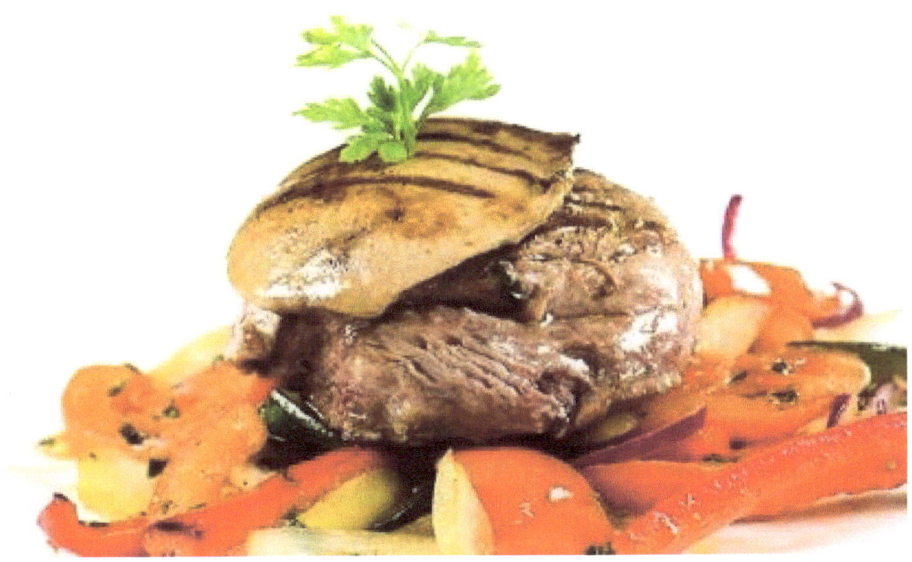

Try reducing on processed foods, especially processed meats and processed cheeses [even though they are so delicious.] These processed foods have lots of salt added to them, so that they do not get spoiled. That is why their shelf life is increased drastically, to up to anywhere between 3 to 6 months after the date of production. Now just imagine eating meat, which has been package 6 months ago, when you could get fresh meat from a farm or from a butcher. Cheeses ripen with age, they say, but would you want to eat something, which has been heavily salted and preserved with chemical preservatives? Instead, look for places, where you can get natural made cheese, with no salt preservatives. Enjoy this cheese and meat. There, you have automatically begun to reduce your intake of salt.

Tips

Also, if you think you are using too much salt in your cooking, try recycling the leftovers, so that you do not need to make fresh dishes with another sprinkling of salt. Any vegetables remaining from previous meals can be used in stews and soups or frozen. Take full advantage of your refrigerator. Even the remaining water, which is normally left over after you have cooked or boiled vegetables can be strained and used as a stock.

Left over nonvegetarian items can be grilled or fried lightly in olive oil, and then served on hot toast. You can also cut them into slivers and strips, and mix them with fresh leafy vegetables and fruit salads. A little bit of rock salt, vinegar, olive oil and a little bit of pepper is going to add to the delicious factor of any dish you prepared with the little bit of care and a little bit of imagination. In fact, these meat pieces can also be put in gravy with a little bit of mint with some chicken stock added and made into sandwich fillings when dry.

If you have some stale bread around, just sprinkle it with water, wrap it up in foil and place it in your oven for a little while. I did not notice whether putting it in the microwave has the same freshening effect on stale bread. You may want to try that out.

 In the same manner, if you have any hotdog buns which have been left over, just cut them into strips, sprinkle with a healthy salt – spice mixture, and then heat them in the oven as toasted bread sticks.

Tasty Salt Spicy Mix

This is a tasty mix, which is normally used as a sprinkle. It is very healthy, because it has spices and other natural ingredients in it. It is also going to have rocksalt/black salt in it, which is much better than processed sodium chloride.

Take six spoonfuls of cumin seed. Place them on the griddle, and stir continuously on a low heat. This cumin seed is going to change color. It is also going to give out a powerful fragrance as it gets roasted. When it turns golden brown in color, remove, allow to cool, and then grind. Place immediately in an airtight glass bottle. This roasted cumin seed is going to be used to add spice to all your dishes, with a little bit of salt and pepper. It is an excellent digestive.

Now, collect together some onion, ginger and garlic flakes – depending on how strong you want their presence in the salt. These flakes are definitely going to lose their power after they have been dried out, when compared to the original. So you can put anywhere between 2 to 3 spoonfuls of each [You are going to learn how to make them in the appendix portion of this book.] Now add for teaspoons each of powdered cinnamon, powdered allspice, powdered cardamoms, coriander seeds, half a teaspoonful of red cayenne pepper, one teaspoonful of black pepper and 2 teaspoons of aniseed to this mixture. You may want to roast all of them – one at a time, please – if you want a really nice and aromatic mixture. Blend together into a fine powder.

Now take 12 teaspoons of powdered rocksalt or 8 teaspoons of powdered black salt. Add this to this mixture, and blend again. Filter and keep grinding until you have a really fine powder.

This is what I call my allspice mixture. Seriously speaking, I cannot do without it, and the amount of this salt, I sprinkle on my food is minimal. So if anybody says that I am eating too much salt, I can just give her the best sneer of my extensive repertoire.

You may want to add   any more herbs, like dried sage, parsley, dried Oregano, bishops Weed, and thyme to this mixture. I keep trying new combinations of different spices, when I am making up this mixture, but I do love the garlic/onion/ginger combination as a base. And of course rocksalt or black salt. The rest of the spices are just to add a healthy and spicy verisimilitude to an otherwise salty narrative.

Using rock salt with onions and garlic in eastern cuisine, is considered to be one of the 1st steps towards good health. Well, we already know that salt is tasty, antiflatulent, and easily absorbed in the body.

 Do you know why Greeks, Spaniards, Italians and the French are comparatively more healthy, when compared to their British counterparts? It is because they do not mind eating garlic and onions, liberally flavored with olive oil, salt, pepper and vinegar with all their meals. This is the reason why they do not suffer much from respiratory, digestive, cardiovascular as well as high cholesterol problems. On the other hand, there are people who are finicky enough to banish these herbs from their cuisine, because according to them, the odour is offensive. In fact, the British called people of these countries "garlic eaters." Well, they may have been rude, but at the same time, they were missing out on all the healthy benefits which they would obtain from these herbs, mixed with olive oil, salt and vinegar as salads.

Do you know that these herbs have some essential nutrients, which are necessary for the proper functioning of the body. So if you cannot bear the thought of them in your daily meal, you may want to take them in some other form, like in garlic pearls or in onion soup. Naturally, this is going to be flavored with rocksalt and pepper.

Appendix

How to make onion flakes

I did not know that one could make onion flakes, really easily right at home, and use them in dishes where you did not want to put in solid onions. These onion flakes would give the dishes a light onion flavor. But living in the East, I got used to the real thing in all my dishes, and I would be really indignant if I went to a restaurant and I found out that the so expensive dish I had just eaten was made up of onion flakes. Nevertheless, it is very easy for you to make onion flakes. These flakes are going to keep anywhere between six months to one year in air tight jars. You can sprinkle them on soups, salads, fillings, or on any dishes which you do not want tasting of the real thing.

Just buy onions in bulk.

Chop the onions into two portions, each or smaller, if you want. Then peel off the layers. You may want to cut the layers into even smaller pieces. If you live in a sunny area, you are lucky, because you can sun dry these onions in the shade. Just place them outside in the sun, cover with a net cloth or a cotton cloth so that those flakes are not subjected to a dust or an insect attack. You are going to find these onions shriveling up and shrinking in size in anywhere between 2 to 6 days. California sun dried tomatoes are shrunk in just this manner. You can try flaking any vegetable you like, including celery.

Once these layers are shrunk, you can either break them up into small pieces with a spoon or with your fingers. If you do not mind your blender, smelling of onions, you can grind them into a powder. And then you can get rid of the smell, by washing out the blender with a handful of solid salt to remove the odor and then rinsing in cold water. Salt is the best cleaning and odor removing material of which you can dream.

How to make Garlic And Ginger Flakes

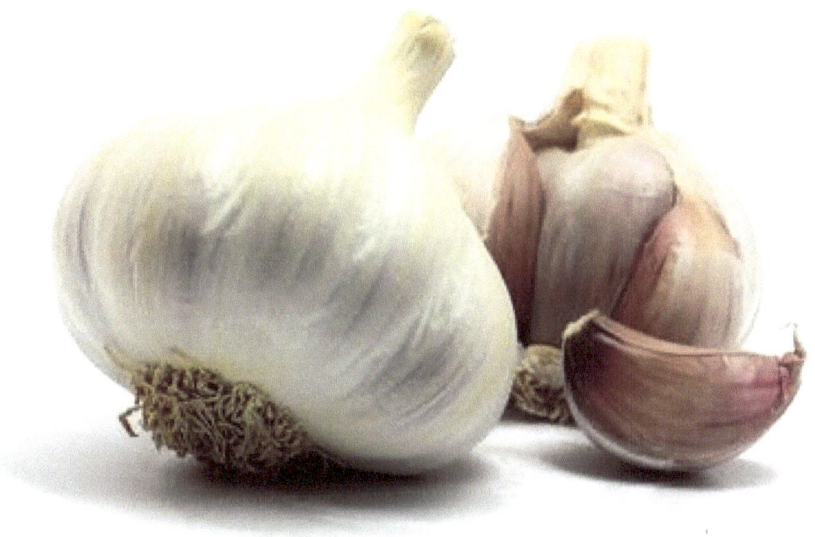

You can make garlic and ginger flakes in the same manner in which I showed you how to make onion flakes. Sun dry them after they have been chopped into small pieces. You may also put them in the oven. Set to the lowest temperature so that they do not burn up. Allow them to dehydrate for about two hours. You can also use a dehydrator to make these flakes.

Desi Ghee

You may have seen an unfamiliar word Desi ghee, in one of the recipes given above.

Desi ghee is just traditional unclarified butter. In fact, I found the best butter to make up Desi ghee was to be found in Denmark under the name of butter- oil. The product in itself was rich, golden in color and delicious to taste. You may also want to look for Irish Kerrygold, which is delicious and pure unsalted butter. Desi ghee is going to be very expensive if you set out to buy it. So make it at home when you have an hour or so, free. This is the ideal cooking fat in the East. It is also used to make up natural medical remedies and also beauty recipes, because after all, it is pure milk. Using it for cooking is a good idea, because it reaches a greater heat than ordinary fats, without burning.

Simmer unsalted butter in a heavy pan. Make sure that they does not burn. This is going to take about 30 minutes. Skim off the upper material floating on the surface, and strain through a Muslin cloth. This quantity is going to reduce by about a quarter, during the heating concentrating process. The end product is the most powerful concentrated healing natural ingredient known to man. Do not use more than one tablespoon to add that extra delicious taste to your food. But if you are preparing meat dishes in this desi ghee, you can use 2 to 3 tablespoons according to the recipes requirements.

You may notice that if you prepare a meat dish in this clarified butter, it is going to separate from the gravy and float on the surface. That is why, you need to stir the gravy again so that the cooking fat gets assimilated in the dish. Even though it looks greasy and oily, the food is definitely not going to taste greasy. That is the best part of cooking in desi ghee.

Conclusion

Now that you know all about the miracle of salt, and how it can be used to keep you healthy, while giving zest to the food you eat, enjoy this gift of nature. Remember, your body needs salt; so the next time you drink fruit juice, just sprinkle some rock salt/black salt and pepper on it.

The only problem with black salt is that it is so addictive that most of the people in the East reach out for it, whenever they want to add that extra zip to all their meals and snacks. On the other hand, professional cooks use it very sparingly, unless of course they are making a highly spicy dish. Instead, they use rock salt. So if you are health conscious and still intend to eat lots of salty delicious stuff, you can use the salt spice mix recipe given here to season your food.

So I am ending this book – with more miracle books to come with a yummy digestive mixture, which is made up very often by grandmas in the East. The yummy tummy mixture is also guaranteed effective to get rid of **gas and flatulence**. Eat a tablespoon after every meal, with a little warm water. However, this is not going to work if you persist on eating greasy, fatty and overly spicy food. Avoid those items in your diet for a couple of days, and try out the appetizer to get rid of your flatulence problems. You can always go back to the Carousel of greasy and spicy food, later on, knowing that you are not going to suffer from constipation, gas, indigestion or any other tummy problems, ever.

Drown hundred grams of Bishops Weed in lemon juice. Dry it in the shade on a sunny day. Now, drown this mixture in horseradish juice. Dry it again in the shade. Now add a teaspoonful each of the following spices – black salt, cumin seed , pepper to this mixture. A couple of teaspoons after every meal will never, ever let you suffer from tummy problems.

Enjoy the magic of salt and look at all of its powerful qualities to heal, in cookery and in beauty.

We have more magic books coming up right here. Enjoy getting to know more about natural remedies and recipes, which help keep you healthy and beautiful naturally.

Author Bio

Dueep Jyot Singh is a Management and IT Professional who managed to gather Postgraduate qualifications in Management and English and Degrees in Science, French and Education while pursuing different enjoyable career options like being an hospital administrator, IT,SEO and HRD Database Manager/ trainer, movie scriptwriter, theatre artiste and public speaker, lecturer in French, Marketing and Advertising, ex-Editor of Hearts On Fire (now known as Solctice) Books Missouri USA, advice columnist and cartoonist, publisher and Aviation School trainer, ex- moderator on Medico.in, banker, student councilor ,travelogue writer … among other things! One fine morning, she decided that she had enough of killing herself by Degrees and went back to her first love -- writing. It's more enjoyable! She already has 48 published academic and 14 fiction- in- different- genre books under her belt.

When she is not designing websites or making Graphic design illustrations for clients ,she is busy browsing in old bookshops for antique books,-she has a mouthwatering collection of priceless First editions and rare books- including R.L. Stevenson, O.Henry, Dornford Yates, Maurice Walsh, C.N.Williamson, Bartimaeus,Oppenheim,Kipling, Sapper De Maupassant, and the crown of her collection- Dickens "The Old Curiosity Shop," and so on- Just call her "Renaissance Woman" - collecting herbal remedies, acting like Universal Helping Hand/Agony Aunt, or escaping to her dear wild forests and mountains for a bit of exploring, collecting herbs and plants, and trekking.

Check out some of the other JD-Biz Publishing books

Gardening Series on Amazon

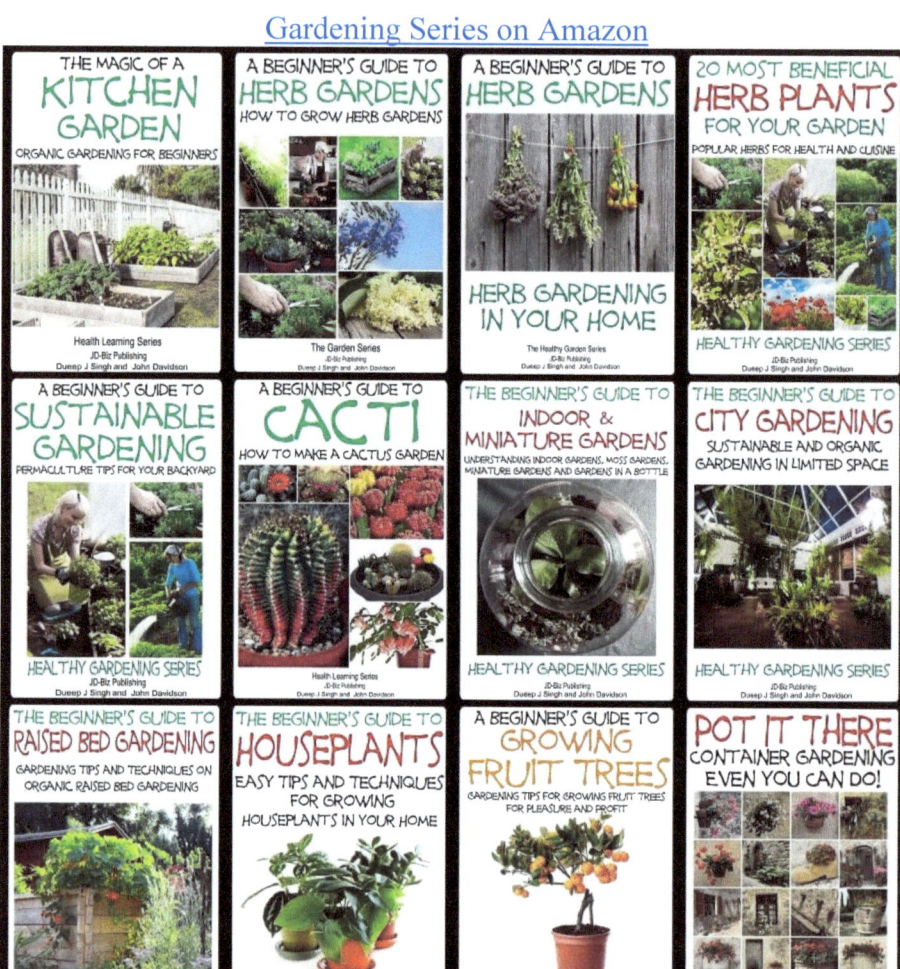

Download Free Books!

http://MendonCottageBooks.com

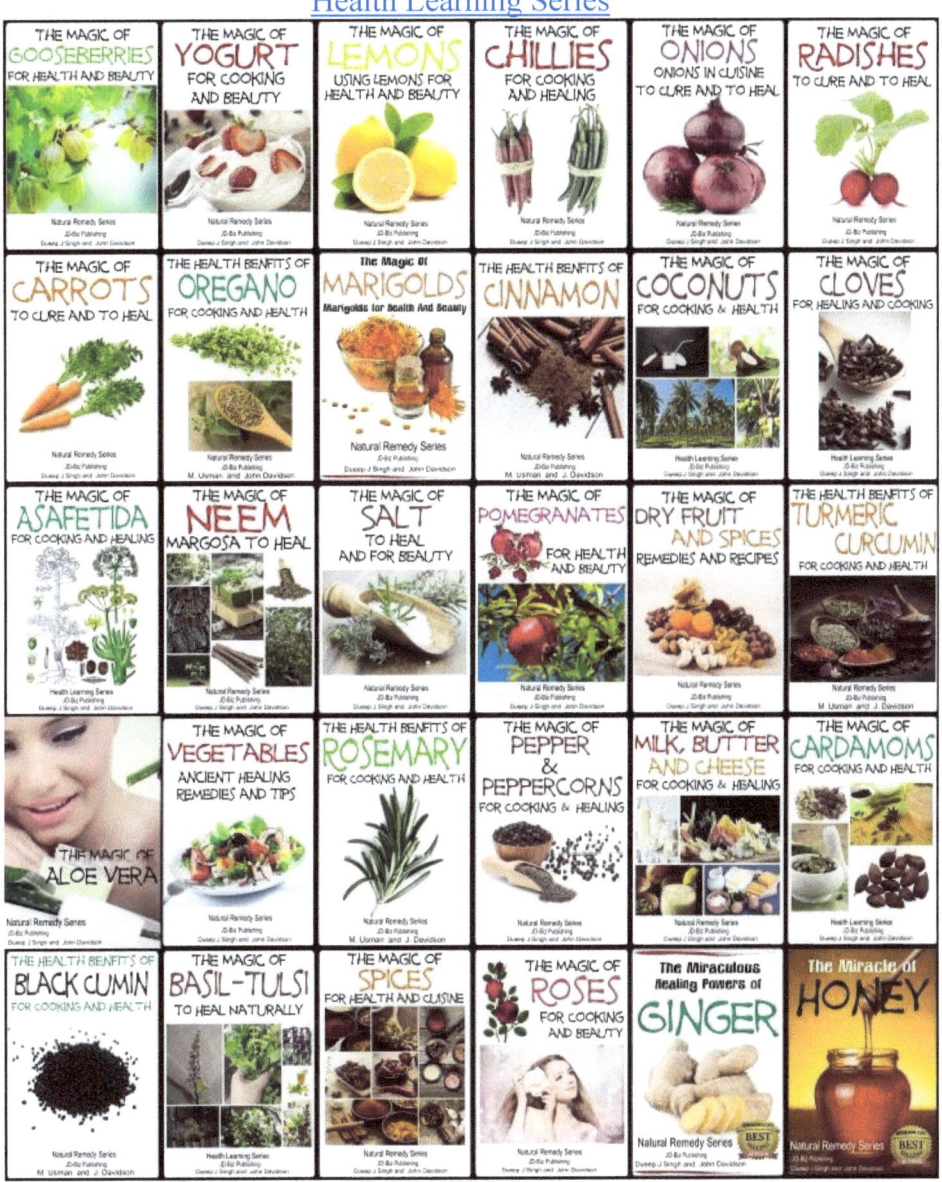

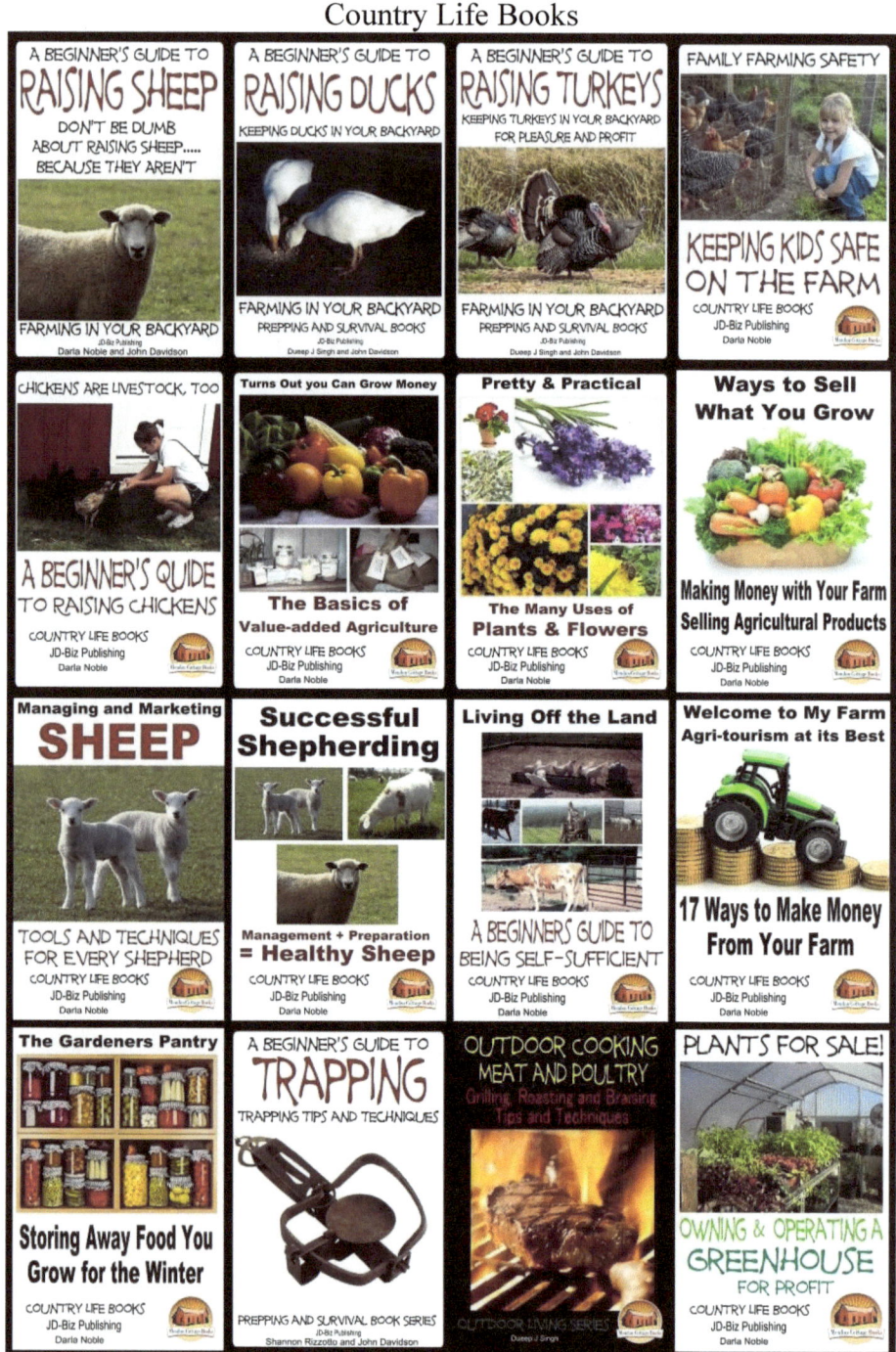

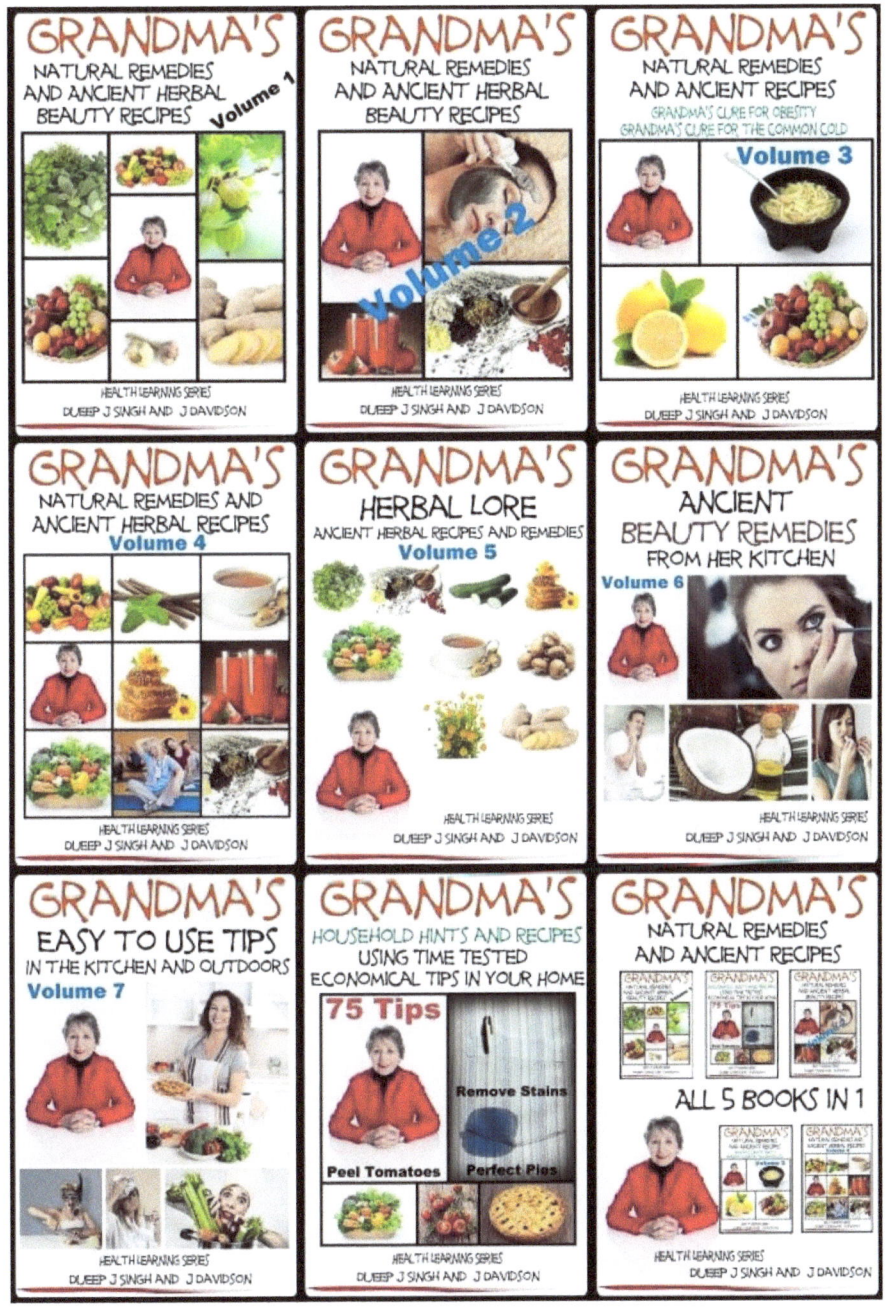

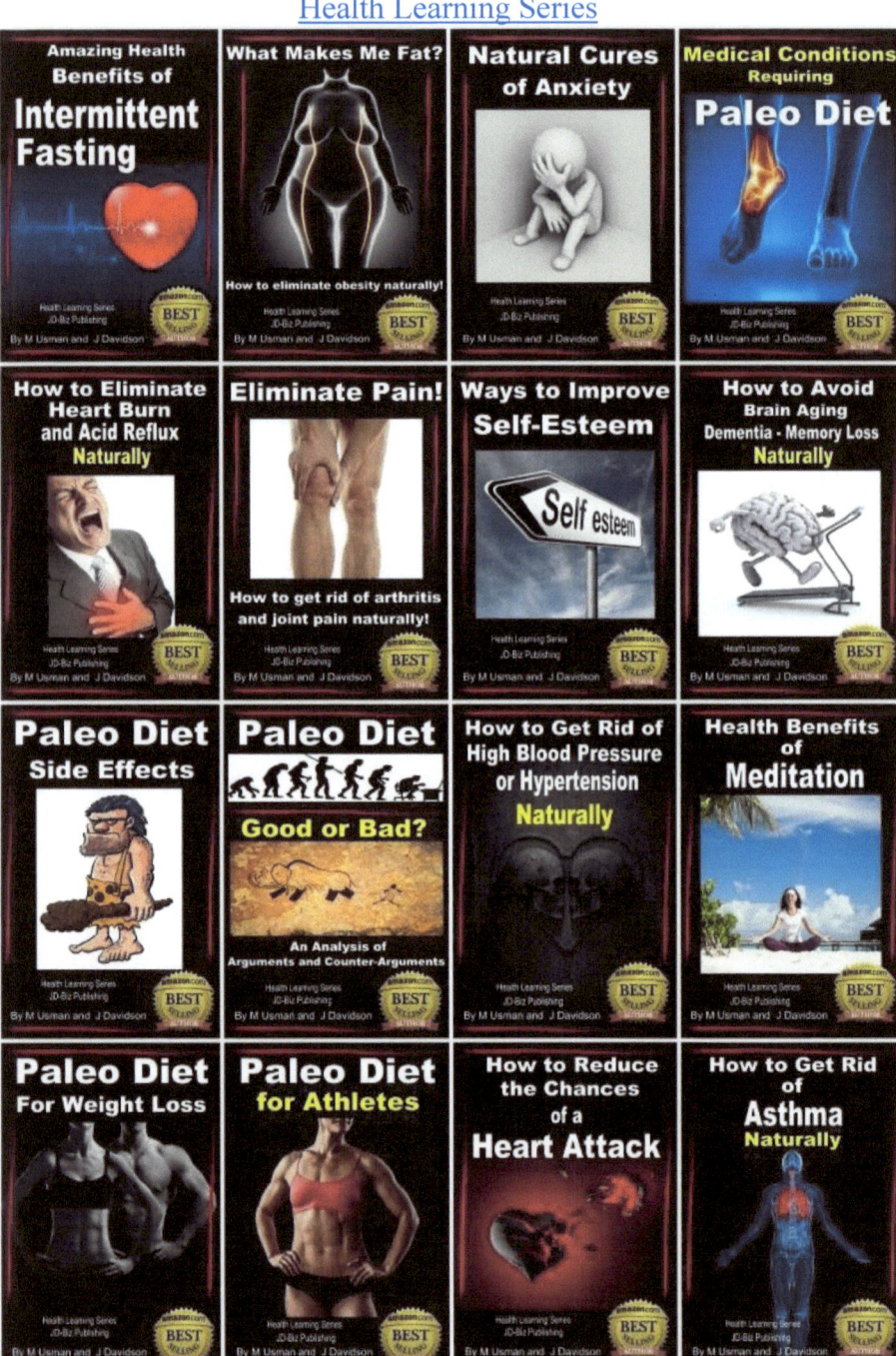

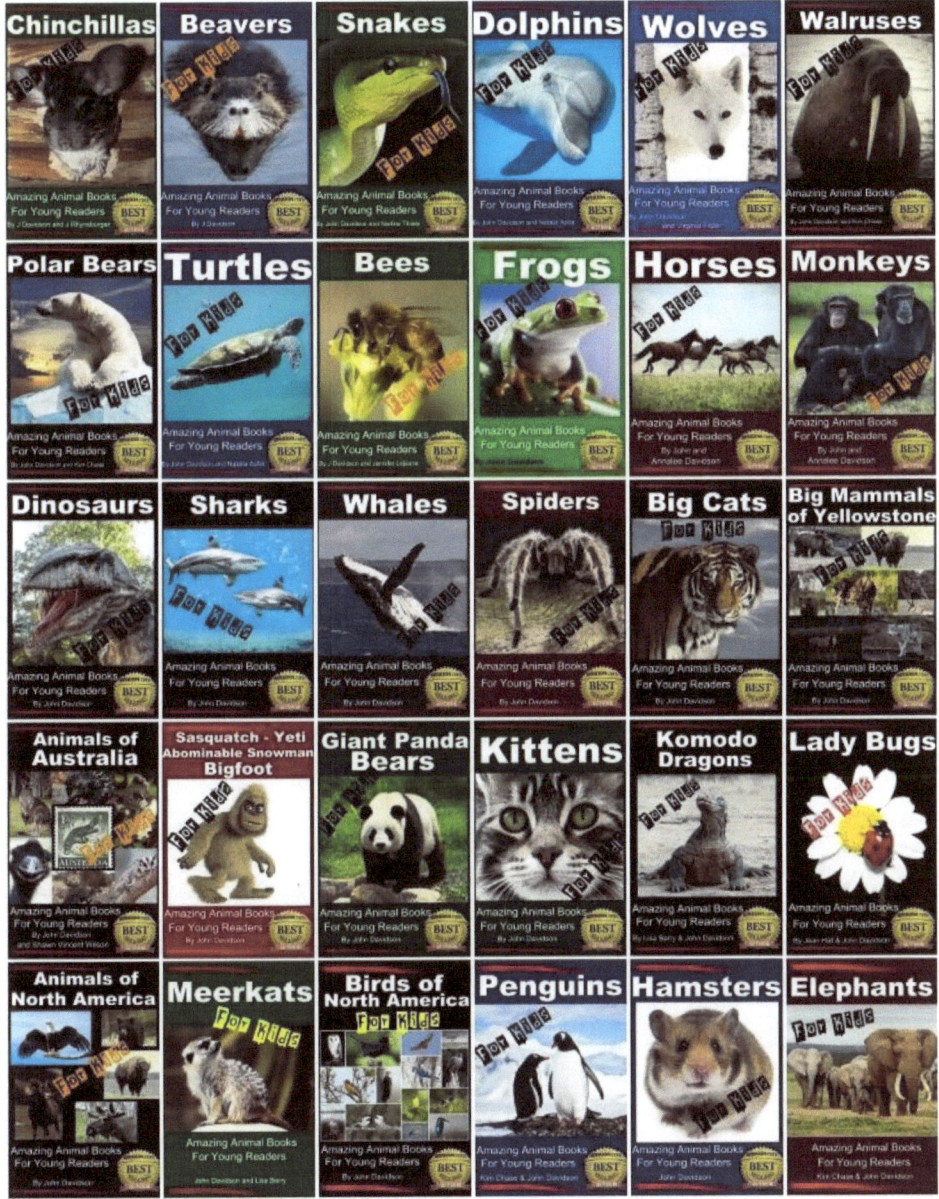

Learn To Draw Series

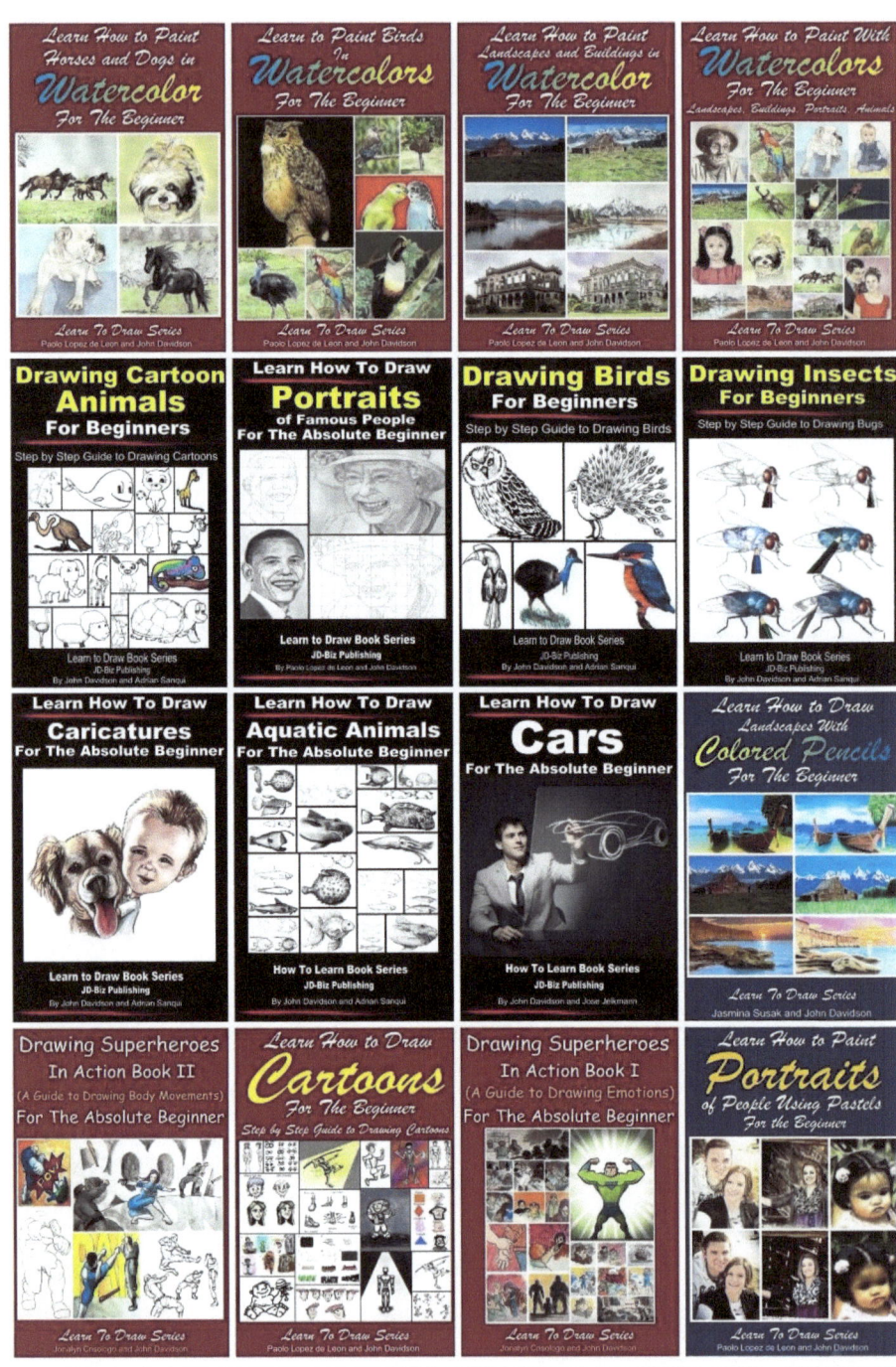

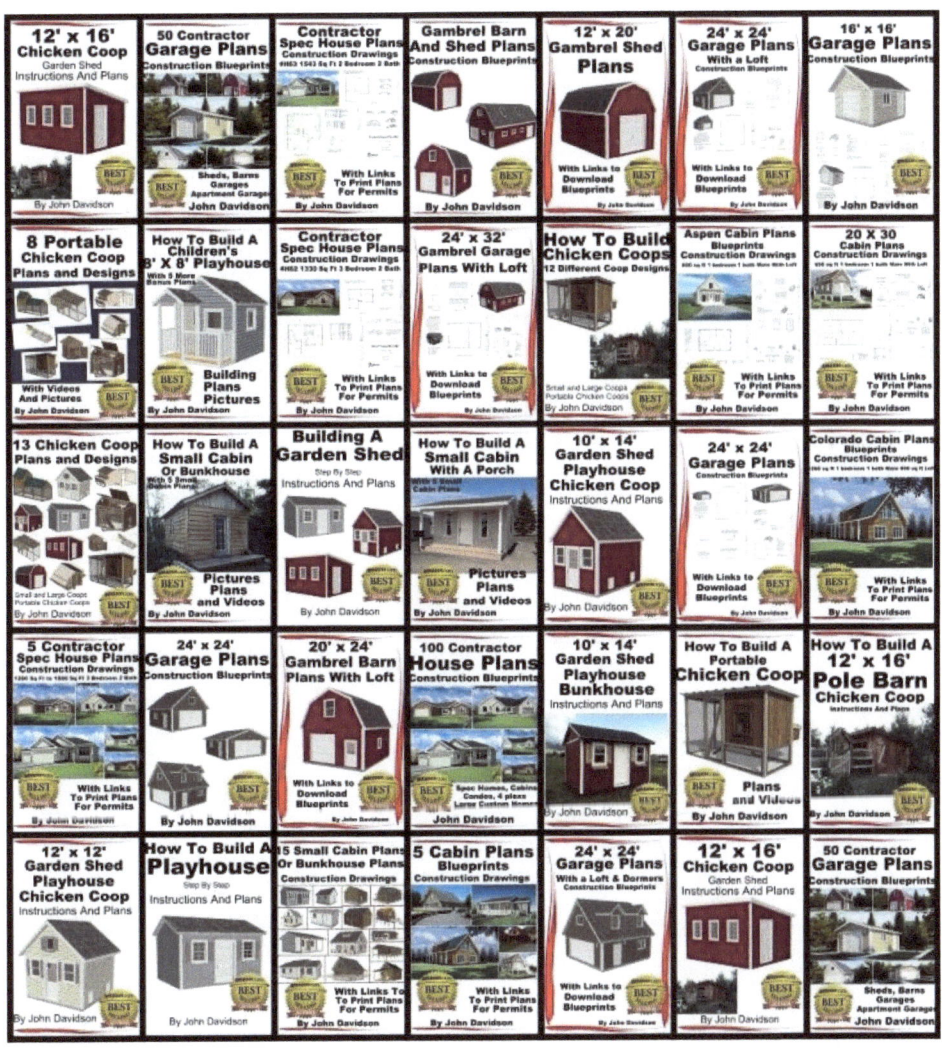

Entrepreneur Book Series

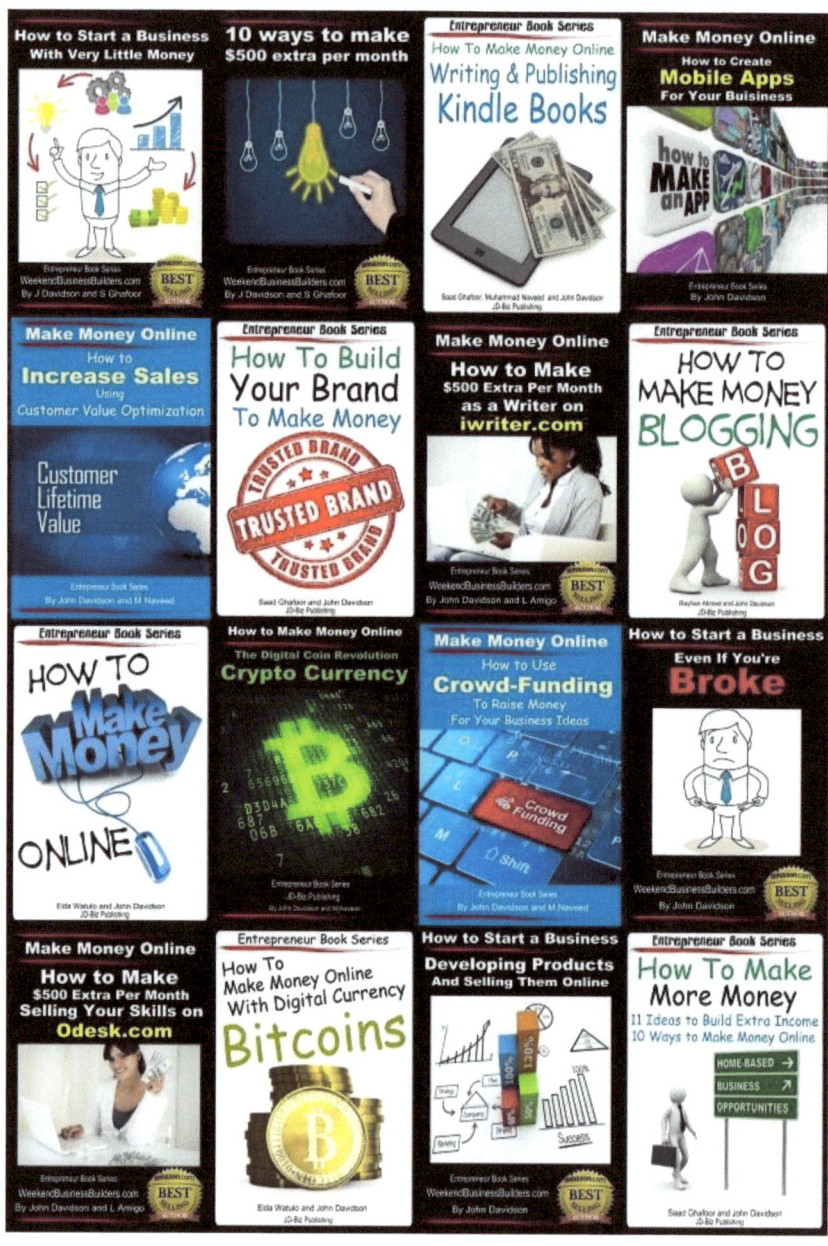

Our books are available at

1. Amazon.com
2. Barnes and Noble
3. Itunes
4. Kobo
5. Smashwords
6. Google Play Books

Download Free Books!

http://MendonCottageBooks.com

Publisher

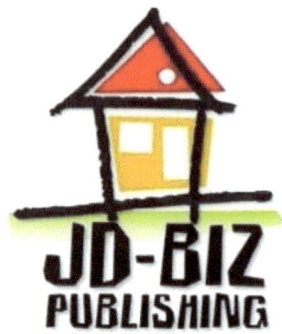

JD-Biz Corp

P O Box 374

Mendon, Utah 84325

http://www.jd-biz.com/

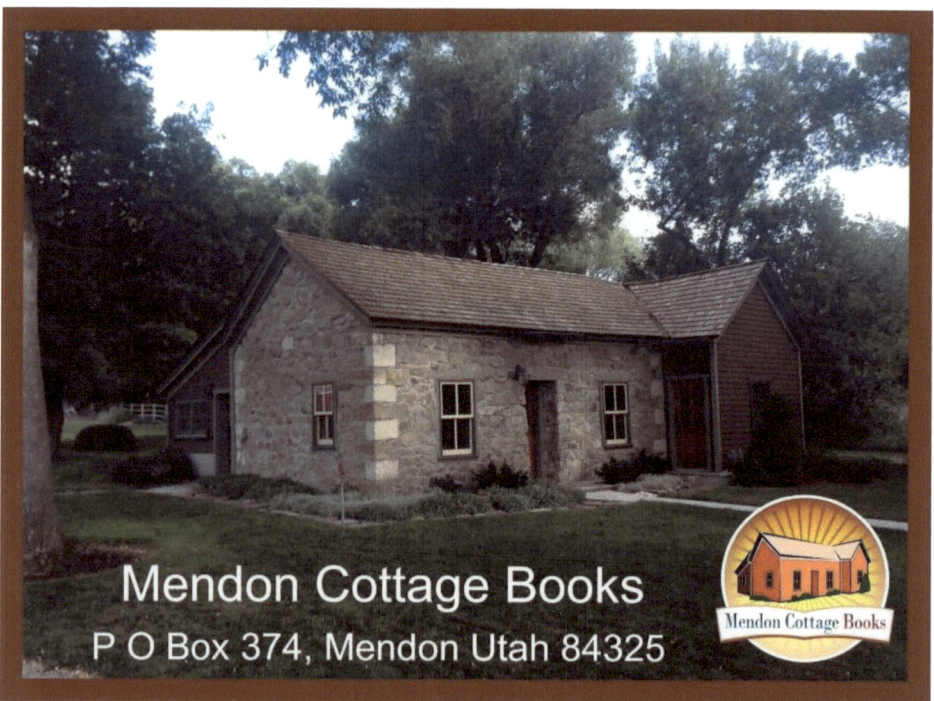

Mendon Cottage Books

P O Box 374, Mendon Utah 84325